shaping
the new
NHS

GOVERNMENT
AND THE NHS –
TIME FOR A NEW
RELATIONSHIP?

STEVE DEWAR

The King's Fund is an independent charitable foundation working for better health, especially in London. We carry out research, policy analysis and development activities, working on our own, in partnerships, and through grants. We are a major resource to people working in health, offering leadership and education courses; seminars and workshops; publications; information and library services; and conference and meeting facilities.

Published by
King's Fund
11–13 Cavendish Square
London W1G oAN
www.kingsfund.org.uk

© King's Fund 2003

Charity registration number: 207401

First published 2003

ISBN 1 85717 481 X

Priced copies available from:

King's Fund Publications
11–13 Cavendish Square
London W1G oAN
Tel: 020 7307 2591
Fax: 020 7307 2801
www.kingsfund.org.uk/publications

Free download available from: www.kingsfund.org.uk/publications

Edited by Alan Dingle
Cover design by Minuche Mazumdar Farrar
Typeset by Kate Green
Printed and bound in Great Britain

Contents

About the author

Foreword   1

Summary   5

Introduction   **8**
Balancing local and national responsibilities   8
Current assessments of the balance   9
Unbounded political accountability   10
The problems with consensus   11
The current position on accountability   12
A future possibility   12

A time for change?   **14**
Safeguarding subsidiarity   14
The nature of political interference   17
Separating accountabilities   21
Executive agency or non-departmental body?   26

A proposal for change   **29**
The agency's role   31
The role of government   36
The role of Parliament   38
Agency governance   41
Domestic and international precedents   42

Conclusion **45**
The historical debate over an NHS agency 46
The case for an NHS agency 48
Ways forward 49

References 51

Linked publications 54

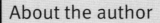

About the author

Steve Dewar
Director of Health Policy, the King's Fund

Steve previously worked in the NHS as a researcher, a public health specialist and a change manager in a district general hospital. Since joining the King's Fund in 1998, he has published widely on the future of the NHS, the development of clinical governance and the regulatory environment that surrounds the delivery of UK health care. His current work includes developing an analysis of health care professionalism.

Foreword

In 2002, our discussion paper *The Future of the NHS* argued that patient choice, provider autonomy and an arm's-length relationship between the NHS and central government could enable health care services to become more responsive, while protecting national standards. In 2003, we have explored these ideas further with discussion papers and linked breakfast debates exploring proposals for expanding patient choice, and considering the role of markets in health care. This paper takes the debate about the shape of a modern NHS a step further.

Since we published *The Future of the NHS,* there have been significant further initiatives to expand choice and provider autonomy. Now it is time, in the words of former NHS Chief Executive Sir Alan Langlands, 'for a serious re-evaluation of the arguments for putting the NHS at arm's length from government' (Langlands 2003). *Government and the NHS – Time for a New Relationship?* considers why such an arm's-length relationship might improve health and health care and explores the case for establishing an NHS agency.

An NHS agency could put politicians and parliamentarians in their rightful and authoritative place, working – in public – to develop and refine health policy. It could bring more transparency to the way the NHS is managed and increase its accountability. It could enable government to broaden its horizons, away from a preoccupation with accountability for each and every action within the NHS, towards a more general concern for the impact of poverty, environment, food, housing and education on health.

The radical step of separating responsibility for developing policy, from responsibility for implementing it, could improve the effectiveness of both activities. It could bring three interrelated benefits: more systematic scrutiny and accountability; a more transparent and inclusive approach to setting expectations for national policy; and greater ownership of targets for improvement by staff in the NHS.

Putting the responsibility for implementing policy at arm's length from government would create a new space between government and those who manage and provide health services. Under the auspices of Parliament this space could be used to construct a system for holding government and the NHS agency to account for their respective responsibilities. Using Parliament as the forum for agreeing the tasks of an agency and the targets for the service would ensure greater openness and more vigorous debate over standards, targets and the impact of policy implementation. This in turn would allow Parliament and the public to focus their scrutiny of government on questions of strategic direction, funding and the coherence, quality and effectiveness of policy.

The high level of public interest in health care means Parliament, political parties, public and media will all continue to debate health care policy and the effect of its implementation. Indeed, debates over what it is right to expect of an NHS agency could ensure a more rigorous and focused approach to policy making and lead to greater consensus over the targets for improvement. When it comes to setting standards and achieving targets, giving an NHS agency responsibility and a voice in the process also offers the possibility of greater ownership by NHS staff of national objectives.

Setting up an NHS agency would mean developing a new system of accountability to scrutinise its work. In effect this would provide better scrutiny of health care policies and their implementation, and opportunities for ensuring expectations for improvement are realistic and command support across the NHS. An agency could be the catalyst for creating this new environment. It could also provide the NHS with the leadership it needs to deliver improvement. Parliament could safeguard these new accountabilities and the resulting responsiveness in the development and implementation of health policy.

In health care, much of the goodwill created by the inclusive approach to devising the NHS Plan has been dissipated, largely because policies have been developed without open debate or collective agreement. The Government now acknowledges the need to re-establish trust and commitment from health service staff. Indeed, recent changes in the Government's approach, such as the establishment of a public service reform forum, are presented as measures to rebuild trust with the unions. This is the context within which a reshaping of the political and management centre of the NHS should be considered.

Establishing an NHS agency does not impose any particular approach to health policy. It could just as easily form part of a strategy that stressed central direction as one that gave more emphasis to local responsibility or the role of a 'managed market'. However, such a change in formal relationships would bring about greater clarity over health policy. For example, consider the way the current down-sizing and reorganisation of the Department of Health presents itself as 'devolutionist' in nature, yet retains a focused (and 'centralist') concern with the detailed outcomes of policy implementation.

Our proposal for an NHS agency would require the minister periodically to put before Parliament a framework defining the boundaries within which the agency should work, its targets and details of its funding. The agency would report at least annually to Parliament and be subject to regular review by parliamentary select committee. Parliament would hold the chief executive to account for the performance of the service.

The idea of an agency has featured in numerous reviews of the NHS structure and organisation, but has never been given serious consideration before. This paper does not analyse every issue that the establishment of an NHS agency might raise. Instead, it explores whether the concept is worthy of wider debate and more detailed analysis both within and outside government.

I hope that you find it stimulating and useful.

Julia Neuberger, Chief Executive

Summary

Government and the NHS – Time for a New Relationship? examines the case for an NHS agency. The idea is not new, but despite repeated expressions of interest in its potential, there has never been a detailed consideration of the case for change, nor an attempt to review its applicability to the current system of health care provision and governance.

The discussion paper considers the conceptual case for an agency in some depth. It:
- examines why national politicians get drawn into local affairs, exploring how the current system of accountability inevitably draws national politicians into managing the operational details of health care delivery
- looks at how to safeguard subsidiarity by creating an effective mixture of local and central responsibilities for improving the health system
- explores the difficulties inherent in dividing accountability between elected and non-elected decision-makers
- compares the advantages of different forms of agency status.

The analysis challenges some of the assumptions that have led previous inquiries, commissions and reviews to reject an agency model for the NHS. It:
- challenges the notion that public sector accountability runs in a direct and hierarchical fashion from individual health provider to Secretary of State for Health
- questions whether it is right that any system of accountability should be judged by how far MPs, and by extension, their constituents, can hold the Secretary of State responsible for any problem or grievance

■ disputes the idea that Parliament only holds ministers to account rather than accepting a broader role in the accountability of civil servants and the chief executives of arm's-length agencies.

The analysis shows what an agency could offer in the context of a health care system increasingly characterised by different forms of arm's-length governance. It concludes that an NHS agency could enable greater parliamentary scrutiny, debate and accountability over government policy-making, the implementation of that policy and the performance of the health system. An agency could also help to improve commitment by NHS staff to the delivery of an agreed set of national standards and targets for long-term improvement.

The paper accepts, however, that these benefits depend on the development of a new understanding of accountability that would keep national politicians at the heart of strategic decisions, while allowing a non-elected agency chief executive to take responsibility for the implementation of policy and subsequent improvement of the health care system. It concludes that parliament would need to be the basis of this new accountability and that it would need to develop its capacity for scrutiny if a 'politically sensitive' agency, at arm's length from government, is to work.

For those who feel that the conceptual challenges to an NHS agency can be overcome, the paper outlines how such an agency might operate. This outline is not intended to be comprehensive, but to encourage policy-makers, politicians and health professionals to engage in debate about the form and structure of such an agency.

This paper envisages an NHS agency that would undertake seven tasks. It would:
■ agree targets for improvement with government
■ allocate funds to the NHS
■ manage performance in line with agreed national targets through existing strategic health authorities

- take a lead on improving NHS organisations (incorporating the work of the Modernisation Agency)
- set clinical standards (and take on the production of national service frameworks)
- co-ordinate national undertakings (such as the NHS programme for research or the development of information and communications technology)
- negotiate national pay.

This 'working model' makes it clear that a proposal for an NHS agency is not about establishing an old-style public corporation, to take over the delivery of health care. It is about reshaping the Department of Health in order to separate policy development from implementation. The agency model builds on the wider experience that politicians and Parliament have of devolved governance in the public services and on a new willingness to consider changing the formal status of civil service departments and NHS bodies to safeguard organisational autonomy alongside national accountability.

Government and the NHS – Time for a New Relationship? calls for wider debate of the agency model and its applicability to health care, particularly among MPs and health professionals, and proposes a formal review, perhaps led by the Cabinet Office, to reconsider the criteria for agency status and their applicability to a possible NHS agency. It also recommends that evidence of good practice should be collected from existing arm's-length bodies to inform policy-makers on how such systems of devolved yet accountable governance could work for the NHS.

Balancing local and national responsibilities

Responsibility for the organisation and management of the NHS has always been divided between the local level and the national level. Local responsibilities have been exercised by individual clinicians and institutions, local commissioners and latterly by cross-institutional clinical networks. National responsibilities have been discharged by the political and managerial centre through a broad range of approaches, from direct 'micro-management' of service delivery through detailed directives, to the setting of standards and more recently the development of an extensive framework of performance targets.

Achieving a mixture that works is central to every NHS reorganisation. Even at the NHS's inception the question of central versus local control took centre stage:

> Parliament has placed the prime responsibility for providing the health services – hospitals, institutions, clinics, domiciliary visiting, and others – on local, rather than central, authority ... To uproot the present system and to put it into the hands of some central authority the direct administration of the new service, transferring to it every institution and every piece of present organisation, would run counter to the whole historical development of the health services ... there is no case for departing generally from the principle of local responsibility, coupled with enough central direction to obtain a coherent and consistent national service.
> (Ministry of Health 1944)

Defining the authority and accountability of decision-making at the local and central levels is a distinctive feature of any government's approach. Indeed, the mixture could be said to define that government's approach. In its second term, the present government has emphasised the twin concepts of national standards and local devolution of decision-making.

Current assessments of the balance

The effectiveness of the current mixture is central to contemporary assessment of the NHS. The Audit Commission review of the implementation of the NHS Plan pointed out the tension between national improvement and the need for local ownership: 'Making more efficient use of resources is an important part of meeting targets and is the key to long-term progress. But for improvement to be sustainable, targets need to make sense locally to encourage strong local ownership of the need to change' (Audit Commission 2003).

Similarly, the Commission for Health Improvement, in this year's first report into the state of the NHS, recognised the value of national targets while at the same time suggesting that they could have a distorting effect:

> *National standards based on national service frameworks or guidance from NICE or the Department of Health are leading to better, more consistent service being available. Waiting times are falling and there are, gradually, more staff available to treat people . . . the concentration on short term waiting targets, which have led to people being seen more quickly, mean that NHS leaders are very stretched keeping the 'show on the road' now, and have limited time for other improvement activities.*
> (Commission for Health Improvement 2003)

Neither of the reports, nor the NHS Chief Executive's annual report into the NHS (Department of Health 2003), have been subject to parliamentary debate or consideration by select committee. Drawing conclusions from the data has, at least publicly, been left to academics, 'think tanks', independent analysts and newspaper columnists.

These assessments, the organisations that produced them and the lack of subsequent debate say three things about the current situation:

- the division of responsibility between 'centre' and 'local' remains central to the current political paradigm for managing public services
- scrutiny is fragmented between different organisations, which results in a bewildering array of reports
- health care scrutiny is rich in reports yet poor in accountability.

Unbounded political accountability

Currently, national politicians are accountable not only for the funding and strategic direction of the NHS, and health care policy, but also for policy implementation and outcome.

Although giving politicians wide-ranging accountability for strategy, policy and outcomes may seem like a good idea, in practice it has mixed consequences. The desire to integrate policy and practice and to ensure demonstrable improvement is well intentioned, but within a complex organisational structure that allocates responsibilities at different levels, through a mixture of local and national decision-making, such centralised accountability strikes a discordant note.

There is a danger that national demands, for which national politicians assume accountability, can limit the scope for local decision-making, and lead to scepticism about the sincerity of national politicians and policy-makers when they claim to respect such decision-making authority. The feeling of being politically manipulated that comes from hearing one policy (local freedoms) and experiencing another (predominant central authority) can lead to disillusionment.

The danger of the current system is that it can restrict the processes of scrutiny, accountability, learning and adaptation. The extent of political accountability for health care can make it hard to acknowledge or publicly respond to criticism (other than in a defensive fashion). It can skew debate, sometimes by depriving it of honest appraisal, sometimes leading to an unwillingness to adapt policy in the light of experience.

Creating independent bodies for assessing the NHS is one part of creating a more open environment. Reshaping the accountabilities of politicians may be another. It could reduce the political risks of debating independent assessments of the NHS, and could enable Parliament to create the space in which this kind of debate can occur. It could bring the realistic assessment of policy out from behind closed doors (where the potential for 'group think' can be high).

The problems with consensus

How far might the involvement of key stakeholders in policy development dilute or enhance government's effectiveness? A more inclusive and open process of scrutiny and debate may require the Government to transfer some degree of influence over policy-making, including input from a wide range of professional stakeholders. This would need to be justified by evidence that their participation had led to better policy and better health care. However, if government engages in such a process but does not cede any influence, those with whom it engages may feel that they are being manipulated to justify decisions already taken.

Listening to people with long (often lifetime) experience of the NHS could enable policy-making to build upon the energies and motivations of the staff who make things happen. However, there may be times when the public expect elected representatives to wield their power against what might be seen as the special interest of powerful employee or professional groupings. This may be where parliamentarians (as distinct from government) have a role. At times, Parliament might need to work with government to hold health care managers, providers and professionals to account – helping to put the public interest before the special interests of any employee or professional group.

The current position on accountability

In a political system that places responsibility for investment, direction, policy, implementation and outcomes at the centre, there can be little sharing of responsibility and credit between national and local decision-makers. This blanket approach to accountability leaves little room for independent assessment to prompt learning and change. This makes the exercise of accountability a relatively crude process. It may also mean that stakeholders (including health care professionals and managers) are insufficiently involved in making and implementing policy. As a consequence, the attempt to achieve consensus, or to align policy with the motivations of health care professionals, is not always made.

In short, the current system of accountability encourages politicians to assume responsibility for all aspects of health policy, creating a situation where there is little room for involving others in a shared process of developing, implementing and evaluating health policy. This restricts the ability of politicians and policy-makers to debate policy openly and to learn about the most effective approach. One response to this problem has been for politicians to create ad hoc advisory committees, policy forums and other groupings of people who have the power, the knowledge or the experience to contribute to the development or implementation of policy. These arrangements have usually been temporary, and the roles, responsibilities and accountabilities of those involved have seldom been clear.

A future possibility

A radical step would be to reshape the political and managerial centre – specifically, the Department of Health – in order to create a more open environment for evaluating national policy and adapting it in the light of experience.

An NHS agency would enable policy-making to be formally separated from policy implementation. It would require the respective roles of central and local decision-makers in health care to be explicitly defined. It would create a space within which Parliament could, with the assistance of others, more effectively scrutinise both service performance and government policy.

Of course, the agency model has disadvantages as well as advantages. So this paper will examine the arguments put forward by the inquiry and review teams who have previously considered the organisation and management of the NHS.

A time for change?

The idea of an arm's-length NHS agency has been considered by numerous inquiries into the structure of the health service. Policy-makers have seen it as offering a better way of organising the complex web of relationships and accountabilities within the NHS.

Do the arguments that prevented people from recommending an NHS agency in the past still apply? Answering this question requires an examination of the historical debate.

With self-conscious pragmatism, the 1979 Royal Commission into the NHS rejected the notion of an agency in favour of a more incremental approach to policy. The commission felt that an agency: '. . . would be necessary only if it became clear that the health departments and authorities could not discharge their responsibilities satisfactorily and that no improvement could be achieved within the existing framework' (Royal Commission on the National Health Service 1979).

The commission went on to conclude that this was 'an important matter about which it is not possible to be categorical at this time, and that it is one that ministers should keep under review'. Almost one-quarter of a century later, the review they envisaged might be considered overdue.

Safeguarding subsidiarity

The National Health Service White Paper of 1944 was 'concerned with the government's proposals for bringing the new comprehensive service into being'. On the question of the appropriate balance between local and central responsibilities, the paper states that 'there is no case for departing generally from the principle of local responsibility, coupled with enough central direction to obtain a coherent and consistent national service' (Ministry of Health 1944).

This analysis is as relevant today as it was in 1944. The 1979 Royal Commission reiterated this position, citing evidence from the government department then responsible for health that 'one of the major concepts on which the present structure of the NHS is based . . . [is] the maximum delegation to Regional and Area Health Authorities of responsibility for providing services in accordance with national policies, objectives and priorities.'

This approach is still a matter of consensus across the political spectrum. The problem is that no government has been able to maintain the approach in a way that all parties involved feel respects the principle of subsidiarity. This was recognised in the 1979 commission and in the 1983 Griffiths Report, which stated: 'The centre is still too much involved in too many of the wrong things and too little involved in some that really matter . . . The Units and the Authorities are being swamped with directives without being given direction' (NHS Management Inquiry 1983).

If the principle of subsidiarity is commonly agreed, it is its achievement that presents a seemingly intractable problem. Two questions need to be asked:

- How would an NHS agency change the way local and national responsibilities are understood?
- Would an agency fit in with current policy as well as being adaptable to any future approach?

If an agency were set up, government ministers and the Department of Health would remain responsible for setting the strategic direction of the NHS – including striking what they believe to be the 'right' balance between national and local responsibilities. This would require an explicit statement of what the principle of subsidiarity meant to the government of the day in relation to health policy and the delivery of health care.

So in response to the first question above, setting up an agency would mean that the Government would have to reveal its views on subsidiary by the act of laying before Parliament a framework for the agency's work – a framework against which both agency and government could be held to account.

In response to the second question, an agency could just as easily fit in with an approach to running the health system that stressed local responsibilities and autonomy as with one that emphasised national direction. Nothing in the agency approach undermines current or proposed reforms. The tension between the budgetary independence and local authority of primary care trusts (and the proposed autonomy of foundation trusts) and national standards and targets would not change with the introduction of an agency. The only difference would be that the profession, the public (through the boards of NHS trusts and the agency) and parliamentarians would have a more explicit role in holding both the agency and the health system to account for acting in accordance with an agreed framework.

Even in 1979 the Royal Commission noted that the lack of formal separation between the roles, responsibilities and accountability of local and national decision-makers encouraged inappropriate 'central involvement':

> It seems to us that the fact that the Secretary of State and his chief official are answerable for the NHS in detail distorts the relationship between the DHSS and health authorities. It encourages central involvement in matters which would be better left to the authorities. In consequence no clear line is drawn where the department's involvement ends.
> (Royal Commission on the National Health Service 1979)

The formal separation of roles implicit in the agency model could create a situation where roles and responsibilities could at least be specified, in the hope that they might be better respected.

The nature of political interference

No government's approach to managing the NHS can ignore the need to change direction. It must be seen to respond to inertia, poor performance, safety problems or sudden political and media focus on a particular case. It is these individual cases that are most likely to impel politicians to take responsibility for detailed aspects of health care, breach the concept of devolved autonomy and take on the mantle of leadership for the organisation – in other words, 'political interference'.

This interference tends to arise when individual cases turn into high-profile political or media events. These cases may be similar in many respects to everyday ones, but for some reason they suddenly become subject to intense media and political examination. Like other extreme events, they are characterised by their intensity and their unpredictability.

Why do these events occur? Individuals, MPs and the media have every right to raise grievances – that is what public accountability means. But how do individual cases become so prominent? One reason may be that they have a personal resonance for all of us. They make us aware that the same thing could have happened to our family, our friends or us.

This awareness may be more effective in shaping public opinion than any number of statistics about the effectiveness of the health system. Statistics are often complicated and their meaning uncertain, whereas a personal story has an immediate and powerful impact. The current expectation that politicians should accept accountability for all aspects of the health services makes it tempting for media and politicians alike to use individual cases of poor (or allegedly poor) treatment as a substitute for more dispassionate analysis. In a system where politics and media relations are full of mutual feedback loops, a 'story' easily becomes the news story of the day. Then, as the story develops a momentum of its own, it takes on symbolic importance – all the parties involved join battle to ensure that their own interpretation of the event becomes uppermost in the public mind.

Whenever the Government's achievement is challenged in this way, the political capital at stake is huge. Ministers and prime ministers face the choice of whether to accept the facts and the meaning ascribed to them, often by others (as in the case of Mavis Skeet, whose cancer became inoperable after repeated cancelled operations) or to dispute the facts (as in the case of Rose Addis, whose family complained of poor treatment in a London hospital).

When interviewed on television by David Frost, Tony Blair used the Mavis Skeet case as an opportunity to announce the Government's intention to raise NHS funding to average European levels. In this way the Prime Minister might be said to have colluded with the notion of individual responsibility, to have agreed the facts and their meaning, and to have used them as a pretext for a significant shift in policy.

> DAVID FROST: *What's your message to Jane Skeet* [Mavis Skeet's daughter] *this morning?*

> TONY BLAIR: *Well, my message is that I accept the responsibility to make sure that the situation that occurred in respect of her mother does not occur, I accept that responsibility, I'm trying to put it right.* (BBC website)

Any incident of this type could become a turning point for individual politicians, parties and administrations. It could scar political consciousness. One only has to think about the exchange between Sharon Storer and Tony Blair during the run-up to the 2001 general election to appreciate how such events can disrupt the presentation of a party's message. When Blair visited a hospital during the election campaign, Storer took out on him the frustration she felt at the way the NHS had treated her husband – and so managed to dominate the media coverage.

The potential impact of such events makes it essential for politicians to have a strategy for managing the risks they bring. Broadly speaking, there are two possibilities: either to attempt to manage the risks from the political centre, or to establish a more subtle notion of accountability that acknowledges the roles and responsibilities of local decision-makers rather than focusing on national politicians. The difficulty with the latter strategy is that the public finds it hard to identify national leadership for health care anywhere other than at the political centre. The concentration of power and accountability for the state of the NHS makes it difficult to reflect the subtleties of a set of responsibilities distributed across a complex system.

The tendency has therefore been to adopt the former strategy: national politicians have tried to show that all that could be done has been done – and in so doing have constantly extended their writ. On the one hand, the public might find it reassuring that national politicians should seek to take responsibility for specific aspects of the health care system. On the other hand, this strategy requires politicians to exercise detailed control over health care (whether through directive, standard or target) in case they find themselves publicly, and politically, accountable for anything that goes awry.

The difficulty with this strategy is that it risks setting up a misleading version of accountability that can obscure the real network of responsibilities. Setting aside for a moment the challenge of imposing political reach over an organisation with the scope and complexity of the NHS, let us look at the simpler issue of accountability within one department of government. The Scott Inquiry into the 'arms to Iraq' affair accepted that:

> *. . . the conduct of government has become so complex and the need for ministerial delegation of responsibilities to and reliance on the advice of officials has become so inevitable as to render unreal the*

> *attaching of blame to a minister simply because something has*
> *gone wrong in the department of which he is in charge.*
> (Riddell 2000)

Superimposing such a system of accountability on a more complex
reality can mean denying respect to local decision-makers. Attempts to
'empower' and motivate managers, commissioners and even public or
patient representatives may fall by the wayside when their authority is
contradicted by a different interpretation of accountability played out
in the national media.

There are times when it may be appropriate for government to take
action at the national level, or to intervene at the local level, because
of a general concern for public safety or because of evidence of local
failure – as with such isolated (and extreme) cases as Rodney Ledward,
Harold Shipman or the practice of organ retention across the country.
But more care should be taken to avoid such interventions when they
are not appropriate.

If there were an NHS agency, Parliament could patrol the boundaries
of accountability and, so long as individual parliamentarians could
set aside party political interests, distribute a proportion of those
accountabilities to agencies and individuals other than government.
Instead of government and media forming the forum in which a spurious
accountability is exercised, the agency model could allow Parliament to
be the arbiter of accountability while respecting the complex reality of
multiple local and central responsibilities.

The high-profile cases cited above are the most obvious examples
of how the political risks created by national politicians exercising
undiluted accountability can lead to a risk management strategy that
emphasises an increasingly centralised approach to health care. By
contrast, an agency might enable the NHS leadership to assume an
appropriate proportion of accountability for the implementation of

policy. This in turn would reduce the political risk for national politicians and allow a greater mixture of local and national responsibilities for the management and organisation of the health system.

If an NHS agency is to be effective in distributing accountability and preventing politicians from being drawn into the detailed business of the NHS, there will have to be changes in behaviour as well as structure. Arm's length governance of how national policy is implemented does not of itself guarantee a more realistic apportioning of credit, blame and accountability. It may, however, provide a suitable foundation for this new approach – 'the permanent and easily identifiable leadership' that the 1979 Royal Commission noted as one of the advantages of an arms-length body (Royal Commission on the National Health Service 1979).

There is one other important consequence of 'political interference' that should be mentioned here. High-profile cases can have damaging effects on the people involved, as they may have to endure a scrutiny of their private lives that they have not invited and for which they may be unprepared. This alone is a good enough reason to reconsider the way in which accountability for events is made the subject of political claim and counterclaim.

Separating accountabilities

The difficulty of distinguishing clearly between the accountability of the agency's chief executive and that of the Secretary of State for Health has often been raised as an objection to an NHS agency. In 1944 the White Paper that prefigured the NHS said of the suggested agency: 'The exact relation of this proposed body to its Minister has never been defined, and it is here that the crux lies' (Ministry of Health 1944).

This type of objection gained support from the criticisms levelled at the prison service in 1995 when Derek Lewis was chief executive and Michael Howard was Secretary of State. Some of those who gave evidence to the public service committee of the time suggested that the problem lay in the political sensitivity of the service at a time of high-profile escapes. It was argued that the prison service was too controversial for agency status, and should be pulled back into its parent departments: '"Making the Prison Service into an agency was", Lord Armstrong told us, "a stage too far"' (House of Commons 1996).

In cases where public service provision is less contentious (for the public or for government), the Committee report suggested that 'the formal delegation of responsibility to agency chief executives can offer better accountability because it makes more transparent the relationship between the minister and the civil servant.' What is more, it concluded that, through the information in the framework document and elsewhere, Parliament and the public may even be 'better able to examine the relationship between Ministers and civil servants to decide to whom should be attributed praise or blame' (House of Commons 1996).

However, this report did not consider an agency to be feasible where the public services in question were politically sensitive. In terms that echo the arguments over the need for politicians to manage risk, the report felt that, in these cases, there were strong pressures on the politician to interfere and strong pressures on agency chief executives to accommodate constantly changing political imperatives. It noted that any simple distinction between policy and operations could be difficult to make because the objectives of the service related directly to individual care. As Lord Armstrong said of the prison service:

So much of the devil lies in the detail of the way in which the individual cases are handled that it is very difficult to maintain this dichotomy between objectives and budgets, on the one hand, and day-to-day management on the other. In a sense the objectives of the agency are so closely related to, and are reflected in the day-to-day actions, that it may not have been a very good case for becoming an agency.
(House of Commons 1996)

The same assertion, that the agency model is unsuitable where the public services in question are politically sensitive, was made by the 1983 Griffiths Inquiry, which felt that an agency would risk formalising 'unnecessarily the role of the corporation vis à vis the secretary of state', something that 'would be extremely difficult in such an intensely politically sensitive operation'. But a closer analysis will show why this blurring of responsibilities might happen for non-statutory agencies and how a different framework for agency status and accountability could work.

A range of organisational forms exists to cater for different degrees of distance between government and service provider. Each form is subtly different from the next, but the main distinction is between those that involve statutory separation and those that remain within their government department and therefore retain the traditional concept of ministerial accountability.

Many agencies exist as separate entities that are nevertheless part of their government departments – a kind of 'half-way house'. They often operate successfully within this framework, particularly where operational matters are easily distinguished from policy matters. Parliament has adapted to this arrangement and increasingly accepts a direct accountability from the agency, with chief executives appearing before select committees and answering parliamentary questions.

In the mid-1990s Sir Robin Butler, the former head of the civil service, argued that it was part of the philosophy of agencies to enable 'a better account directly from the Chief Executive than from the Minister', but he added the important caveat that 'if Parliament is then dissatisfied with that, or an MP is dissatisfied with that, that MP always has the right to go to the Minister and ask the Minister to intervene.' A similar desire to ensure that MPs retained the right to raise matters of importance to their constituents 'directly with the minister responsible' informed the 1979 Royal Commission's rejection of the agency model.

It may not be possible to introduce genuine subsidiarity into the
organisation of health care by setting up a formal arm's-length body
and at the same time to preserve the right of appeal to a minister over
any issue. Given the myriad alternative routes for accountability – via
agency chief executive, select committee and grievance procedures as
far as the health service or parliamentary ombudsman – the agency
model offers considerable advantages over this right of appeal.
This spurious ministerial accountability now has little more than
symbolic value.

As we have seen, problems arise with the current arrangements for
accountability when the service is politically sensitive. Ministers then
feel obliged to take responsibility for operational detail – just in case
they find themselves answering to a dissatisfied Parliament or a
dissatisfied MP.

Managing the party political risk and the personal risk to their
ministerial career means keeping an eye on the many operational
matters that might suddenly become 'politically sensitive'. As a result,
any agency arrangement that does not change the underlying
accountability (such as a 'half-way house' arrangement) is unlikely
to work in an area such as health. It would not be realistic to specify
a framework that gave an agency chief executive sufficient freedom
to manage the NHS if a minister remained immediately answerable for
every operational detail.

A tacit acceptance by Parliament that an agency chief executive is
accountable for operational matters is not enough. A more formal
separation is needed – such as the creation of a separate statutory
NHS agency. Indeed, Derek Lewis himself advocated this as a solution
to the problems of confused responsibility that afflicted the prison
service in the mid-1990s.

Statutory independence might be seen as a means of reducing the ability of a Minister to interfere in the work of the agency. Derek Lewis described a possible arrangement for the Prison Service in which agencies were non-departmental public bodies within a statutory framework . . . The Service would be overseen by an independent board established by statute; policy would be set by Ministers through secondary legislation; and funding levels would be determined by the sponsoring department; and the sponsoring department would monitor efficiency through 'systematic and rigorous performance audits conducted by an independent inspectorate' . . . One of the benefits of such an arrangement, according to Mr Lewis, would be that Ministers were no longer responsible for the operation of the Service: 'It would put greater distance between the sponsoring department and the Chief Executive and would provide the Chief Executive with some reassurance against the doubtless unnecessary fears that expressing unpopular views might bring swift retribution.'
(House of Commons 1996)

A formally separate NHS agency would allow such a new system of accountability to develop. The agency's chief executive would become directly accountable to Parliament for the work of the agency. A statutory relationship would mean government setting down what it requires of the NHS agency and seeking approval from Parliament – thus enhancing parliamentary input into the policy process. Ministers would still have powers to appoint and dismiss the agency's chief executive. However, there would not be the same recourse to the minister if Parliament or an MP were dissatisfied, unless there was an issue of national policy or public safety at stake or the agency was failing to live up to the performance framework set by Parliament.

Executive agency or non-departmental body?

In 1944 the White Paper that preceded the foundation of the NHS considered two versions of the agency model. The first was of an agency or corporation where, in conformity with traditional practice, the ultimate responsibility rested 'with a Minister of the Crown, answerable directly to Parliament and through Parliament to the people' – in other words, the 'half-way house' or executive agency solution.

In 1983 the Griffiths Inquiry called for what was effectively an informal version of an executive agency board – a small, strong, professional management group that included a general manager vested with authority. Such an arrangement could, it was claimed, ensure 'that the statutorily appointed authorities manage the NHS effectively' and therefore the appointment 'would leave undisturbed your [the Secretary of State's] clear responsibility for overall policy direction and for the handling of the public and political sensitivities of the service.'

Griffiths was seeking an effective, if informal, separation between NHS central management and political responsibility for national policy. It was also an attempt to limit the activities of the centre so that day-to-day NHS management could rest with local decision-makers. Griffiths, however, recommended this approach without calling for changes in the formal relationships between national politicians, the Department of Health and local NHS organisations, changes in the accountabilities of the minister or a formal separation between politicians and national management. The resulting management board did not last. This confirmed the conclusion of the 1944 White Paper that this type of arrangement offered no advantages as it did not change the current accountability of the minister.

Central responsibility must rest with a Minister of the Crown, answerable directly to Parliament and through Parliament to the people. The suggestion has been made that, while this principle

should be accepted, there is a case for replacing the normal
departmental machinery by some specially constituted corporation
or similar body . . . which would, under the general auspices of a
Minister, direct and supervise the service. The exact relation of this
proposed body to its Minister has never been defined, and it is here
that the crux lies. If in matters both of principle and detail decision
normally rested in the last resort with the Minister, the body would in
effect be a new department of Government . . . If, on the other hand,
certain decisions were removed from the jurisdiction of the Minister
(and consequently from direct Parliamentary control) there would be
a need to define with the utmost precision what these decisions
were. Clearly they could not include major questions of finance.
Nor could any local government authorities responsible for local
planning or administration reasonably be asked to submit to being
over-ruled by a body not answerable to Parliament.
(Ministry of Health 1944)

The second, more radical option – removing certain decisions from 'the
jurisdiction of the Minister' – was also considered by the 1944 White
Paper. Although the assumptions on which its analysis was based were
sound for the time, it is worth reconsidering them from the viewpoint
of today. For example, the claim that if decisions were taken out of the
'jurisdiction' of the minister, Parliament could not hold the new
decision-maker to account is questionable in the light of more recent
experience. Since 1944 hundreds of organisations at arm's length from
government have been created to provide, manage or regulate public
services and public expenditure. Of these, 192 are executive non-
departmental public bodies (NDPBs) – the form that we recommend
for the new NHS agency. Ten of the existing executive NDPBs (such as
the Commission for Health Improvement, the Human Fertilisation and
Embryology Authority and the Commission for Patient and Public
Involvement) are already sponsored by the Department of Health, and
employ more staff – a total of 4,000 plus – than the department itself.

Accountability arrangements have been developed for these statutory separate entities, and Parliament and ministers now accept the need to distribute areas of responsibility between the minister and the chief executives. Through the agreed frameworks that specify their role, agency chief executives are regularly (although not systematically) called to account by select committees, regularly respond to parliamentary questions, and their organisations present their decisions and actions to the public through the media. Taking decisions out of the 'jurisdiction' of the minister no longer means excluding Parliament from exercising a scrutiny and accountability function in relation to the new body. Indeed, agency status and the development of parliamentary roles may between them result in greater accountability than the tradition of holding ministers to account.

The NHS and the Department of Health are in many ways an exception to a contemporary rule of increasingly devolved governance for public services. In an area as politically sensitive as health a real separation of roles and responsibilities would require an agency based on the Non-Departmental Public Body model. This would ensure that politicians could not be pulled back into assuming day to day responsibility for agency business. The 1944 White Paper is right to highlight the consequential problem of specifying the exact areas of agency responsibility – but the process of establishing this specification may, under parliamentary and public scrutiny, bring higher levels of ownership for future direction amongst NHS staff, a more realistic approach to setting targets for improvement and a higher level of scrutiny over subsequent performance.

A proposal for change

There has long been interest in how far the agency model is applicable to health care. Yet no review of the NHS has ever got beyond the conceptual challenges to current models of organisation and outlined the possible arrangements for an NHS agency. This paper has looked at those conceptual issues and, it is hoped, demonstrated that traditional objections to the agency approach can be legitimately challenged. This section of the paper will therefore make proposals about the possible functions, governance, accountability and precedence of an NHS agency.

The approach will be illustrative rather than comprehensive, providing enough detail to show how an agency might work. The aim is to stimulate debate over such questions as why an agency should take on this role or that task, why it should have a board modelled on this rather than that type of organisation, and so on.

The precise specification of an NHS agency could provoke passionate debate, but our aim has been to open up discussion about how an agency could fit without major disruption into the current changing health care environment. As a starting point, Figure 1 (overleaf) summarises the proposed relationships and roles for government (Secretary of State and Department of Health), agency and Parliament at the heart of this proposal.

FIGURE 1: Respective accountabilities and respective roles

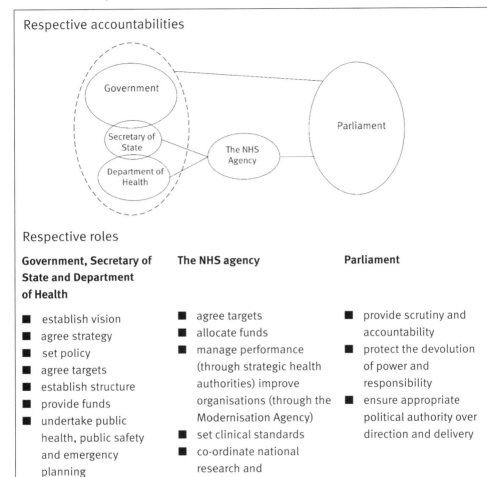

Respective accountabilities

Respective roles

Government, Secretary of State and Department of Health	The NHS agency	Parliament
■ establish vision ■ agree strategy ■ set policy ■ agree targets ■ establish structure ■ provide funds ■ undertake public health, public safety and emergency planning	■ agree targets ■ allocate funds ■ manage performance (through strategic health authorities) improve organisations (through the Modernisation Agency) ■ set clinical standards ■ co-ordinate national research and development/information and communication technology ■ negotiate pay frameworks	■ provide scrutiny and accountability ■ protect the devolution of power and responsibility ■ ensure appropriate political authority over direction and delivery

(King's Fund 2003)

The agency's role

An NHS agency could undertake the following seven major roles:

■ Agree performance targets with government

Two sets of targets need to be agreed with government and Parliament.

The first set is comprised of those that specify the agency's role and establish indicators of effectiveness against which Parliament and the minister can hold the agency, its chief executive and its board accountable.

The second set is those targets that apply to improvement in the NHS, whether specified in terms of policy implementation or health outcomes. Some of these targets are currently determined as part of the Department of Health's negotiations with the Treasury and are set out in the department's public service agreement. Adopting an agency model would mean that other parties could be involved in the negotiations, potentially giving the targets wider acceptance and ownership.

An NHS agency would make it possible to include a range of stakeholders. Members of the public or patients could serve on the board, and people with experience of policy implementation could become members of the executive team. Whether it also involved professional bodies would be up to the agency.

By introducing the formal separation of government and agency, Parliament inherits the important role of ensuring that targets express democratically mandated expectations for the NHS while at the same time tempering political ambitions with objections from wider stakeholders. Because of its parallel engagement in the processes of scrutiny and accountability, Parliament could over time bring considerable experience to bear on this task.

■ Allocate national funding

Critics may ask, 'Is it right that Parliament should raise funds and an agency allocate them?' This paper proposes an alternative: that Parliament and government should hold an agency to account for its use of public money.

If an NHS agency is to assume responsibility for implementing national policy and improving the NHS, it should have a role in the allocation of funding. Targeted financial resources and financial incentives need to be available to those who are going to be held accountable for policy implementation and improvement.

The roles of agreeing targets and funding their implementation will need to remain connected. An agency will have to develop its authority and credibility by ensuring that national standards and targets are costed and achievable. This could be important for engaging the commitment of health service staff and building trust between the agency, staff and the wider public.

However, the same argument does not necessarily apply to all financial allocations (many of which are determined by a complex formula reflecting political considerations). Capital allocations may, for example, be a case in point. The agency's accountability for national targets and its ability to allocate money for implementation and improvement should certainly be linked, but how far the agency, rather than the Department of Health, should be responsible for allocating other elements of NHS funding would need to be debated by a wider (and technically informed) group.

■ **Manage performance through the strategic health authorities (directly accountable to 'the agency')**

Responsibility for strategic health authorities would be a necessary precondition for an agency to accept the remit to manage the implementation of national policy across the NHS. It is worth noting that, even with an agency model, the tension between national direction and local responsiveness remains. The need to connect national policy with the implementation of that policy in more locally based organisations is incontrovertible. Allowance must also be made for an established agency to develop into a more regional structure if the political will for regional devolution takes hold.

■ **Lead organisational improvement across the English health service, including direct responsibility for the functions currently undertaken by the Modernisation Agency**

Bodies that report on NHS performance should remain independent of an agency that will be held accountable for improvement. Therefore organisations such the Commission for Health Improvement (or the proposed Commission for Health Audit and Inspection) and the proposed regulator for foundation trusts should remain independent of the NHS agency, and should have their own direct accountability to Parliament. This will help Parliament to bring together the evidence from the various organisations that scrutinise the achievements of the agency and the health system – thus enabling Parliament to hold agency and government to account for policy and implementation respectively.

However, the organisations involved in developing staff and setting national clinical standards (the Modernisation Agency, the National

Health Service University and possibly the National Institute for Clinical Excellence – see below) could either be incorporated into an NHS agency or be made accountable to it. This would help solve the problem of the unco-ordinated proliferation of national agencies in health care. A variation of this approach would be to put these organisations at arm's length from the NHS agency, which would be their co-ordinating or sponsoring department. This arrangement would:

– minimise the disruption of existing organisational boundaries and structures

– keep the organisations concerned focused on delivering their highly specialised services

– but still bring a degree of co-ordination to the task of implementing national policy.

■ **Set clinical standards – managing the process of developing national service frameworks and implementing National Institute of Clinical Excellence recommendations**

Setting and updating clinical standards – which includes ensuring that services are consistent across the country – has major resource implications. Since politicians are responsible for NHS funding, such standards should be subject to debate in Parliament. This might be particularly appropriate when they also raise ethical issues, such as any extension of the availability of IVF treatment.

This debate could form part of a dynamic process whereby expectations for service improvement or implementation are agreed and responsibility is passed to an NHS agency. The real opportunity cost of the measures proposed should be fully discussed before they go forward for implementation.

It can be argued that NICE is an encouraging organisational precedent for an NHS agency – it certainly demonstrates the ability of an arm's-length agency to effectively handle politically sensitive issues. Although its work is not without critics, it has undertaken its job without any collapse in public, professional or political confidence. However, the case for agency status rests on the potential to enhance accountability as much as the possibility of obtaining improved effectiveness – however that may be defined. When it comes to setting managerial priorities for the service as a whole, the work of NICE (as much as the work of any agency) should be subject to robust political accountability, and its decisions considered in the round when it comes to setting managerial priorities for the service as a whole.

This could be achieved by an NHS agency feeding the proposals from the National Institute for Clinical Excellence (NICE) into a routine round of debate with the Department of Health, the Secretary of State and the Treasury, as well as with Parliament. Alternatively, proposals (from NICE) could go directly to the Department of Health and then into debate with the Treasury, the agency and Parliament. It is a moot point which is the better route. However, this arrangement could ensure that NICE's recommendations are discussed in a wider forum before being adopted, at which point the agency assumes responsibility for implementation.

■ **Co-ordinate a national approach to research and development and the development of information and communication technology**

How should such functions as research and development (R&D) and information and communication technology (ICT) be co-ordinated, or even centrally controlled? An NHS agency could have a role here, but the issue would need to be widely debated first. For example, it could be argued that, since health R&D should cover non-NHS as well as NHS activity, and since most of its public funding is not spent within the NHS, a national NHS agency should not determine a national approach. On the other hand, there is also a case for bringing a strong centralising force to bear on a regional structure that can militate against co-ordinated action and national standards. Similarly, there is vigorous debate over the best approach to ICT and the relative effectiveness of central specification versus local freedom. An agency model would require a clear policy to be adopted, and the case to be made for working within or outside the agency.

■ Negotiate national pay

Although the introduction of an NHS agency might affect current arrangements for negotiating national pay, this proposal is not intended to skew current debate over pay bargaining or to resolve questions about the place of other bodies in the machinery used to negotiate pay.

However, two points are worth making here. First, whenever there is a pay dispute there will always be a role for national politicians in resolving claims against national resources. Second, it could be that in discussions over national pay, an NHS agency could appropriately fulfil the 'principal employer' role.

The role of government

Within this structure, the government, the Secretary of State and the Department of Health would establish the vision for the NHS and work with the agency to:

- provide funds, setting the direction for the private finance initiative, the financial framework for capital allocation or the financial systems for hospital payments
- set the strategic direction, including such areas as the extension of patient choice, and agree policy and improvement targets
- establish the structural framework for the delivery of health care and shape the broader regulatory environment for health services (using legislation where appropriate)
- lead on public health, public safety and emergency planning
- co-ordinate policy development across department, sectors and counties.

Much of the Government's role would require continuous dialogue between the Department of Health and the agency, for issues as varied as establishing principles to guide the future development of PCTs or strategic health authorities; work to revise and approve a new NHS Plan; or establish new plans for particular services, such as intensive care, or particular disease areas such as cancer. The key to understanding the Government's role working with an NHS agency is the need for it to engage in discussion, negotiation and agreement over future plans.

There is nothing to stop departments and arm's-length bodies from working together. Setting public service agreements could be a case in point. Here, the Office of Public Services Reform, in its review of public bodies, has already concluded that:

> . . . *departments and agencies must together ensure that agency targets are real, challenging and responsive to customers. Departmental and agency target-setting must be aligned and timetabled to support Public Service Agreements and be supported by spending decisions. Key service delivers should be fully involved in setting targets in Spending Reviews.*
> (Office of Public Services Reform 2002)

Current arrangements raise legitimate concerns that issues of public health are being obscured by the focus on health service performance. An agency model would also enable governments to consider the way in which it might intervene to improve the impact on health of national income, environment, food, housing and education.

Establishing an NHS agency offers the Government and Department of Health a broader role in relation to health, and a narrower (but more effective) role in relation to health care. It creates an opportunity to create an actual department *for health* that could even extend its remit to some of the roles of other departments with a substantial impact on health.

It also enables the Government and Department of Health to recast itself in the role of 'funder' or 'purchaser' of health care, working at a distance from those with the responsibility for managing the provision of health care (either directly or indirectly, in the agency, strategic health authorities and PCTs). Government could then take the opportunity to work with Parliament and independent regulators to identify and require changes in policy and direction.

A new Department of Health could request a response from an NHS agency to high quality audit and scrutiny and, if necessary, even impose sanctions upon an agency. Having taken itself out of the politically dangerous position of having to respond itself to each and every criticism made by inspection, committee report or evaluation, it could apply its democratic authority to the task of ensuring or enforcing action from those with a more real accountability for services.

Historically, departments exercising sponsorship roles in relation to arm's-length agencies have not had this sort of access to the high quality independent regulation and assessment that the Commission for Health Improvement (CHI) and its proposed successor the Commission for Health Audit and Inspection (CHAI) – among others – could now provide. This makes a real difference to the case for an NHS agency. It allows for agency status to be seen as part of a division of roles that could be discharged in the sort of informed environment that might enable an effective and meaningful accountability for respective roles and responsibilities to emerge.

The role of Parliament

Parliament would agree the framework for the agency's work and the standards and targets it would seek to implement across the NHS. Parliament would also receive from the independent regulators the assessments of performance against these frameworks.

This would put Parliament at the apex of accountability, empowering it to hold the Government to account for funding, strategic direction and policy coherence, and the agency alongside NHS to account for the implementation of policy.

On occasion, Parliament may need to act to protect the devolution of power and responsibility to an agency and to more autonomous health care providers. On other occasions it might need to lend its authority to efforts to establish a new strategic direction or to hold service providers to account for delivery.

Parliament already uses the Health Select Committee and the Public Accounts Committee to hold the NHS to account. These are good – if limited – parliamentary resources usually conducting detailed scrutiny over well-defined areas of health interest, often out of the public spotlight. The development of an NHS agency may require a more substantial architecture of parliamentary input and scrutiny.

Essentially, this architecture would need to integrate regular and systematic scrutiny (through a powerful committee) with parliamentary debate. Key and recurring topics would need to include:

- considering the annual independent assessment of NHS performance – something that attracted little parliamentary time in 2003
- a regular review of the opportunity costs for clinical standards (encompassing the decisions made by the NICE)
- the agreement of a periodic framework for NHS agency work. This would cover a specified period and would include objectives for the agency and national standards and targets for the NHS (to be implemented through the agency).

It is particularly important that an NHS agency chief executive should have authority and credibility with the public. To a large degree this will rest on the status that they are given by politicians and the media alike. To be accepted as the voice of the NHS on Radio 4's Today programme requires that they are accepted as the voice of the NHS within Parliament. This would require a change of parliamentary perspective on the NHS, and Parliament may have to be creative about how it goes about its own reform. Its objectives should include ensuring an increased ability:

■ to scrutinise policy and performance
■ to expose to debate issues of public expectation and cost
■ to hold multiple actors to account for the organisation, management and delivery of public services.

The growth of agencies was recognised by the Hansard Society Commission on Parliamentary Scrutiny (2001) as 'both a challenge and an opportunity for Parliament'. *The Challenge for Parliament* sets out how a reformed Parliament might work, 'drawing more effectively on the investigations of outside regulators and commissions, enhancing the status of select committees and clarifying the role of Parliament and its politicians.' Implementing the commission's recommendations could help create the effective parliamentary scrutiny that is so central to the agency proposal.

Hansard Society Commission on Parliamentary Scrutiny

The seven central principles for reform are:

1. Parliament at the apex
'Recommendations aim to create a more formal and organised relationship between those outside bodies and Parliament, to promote more systematic scrutiny by both the Commons and the Lords.'

2. Parliament must develop a culture of scrutiny
'Party loyalties and demands need to be balanced with scrutinising
the executive and holding government to account.'

3. Committees should play a more influential role within Parliament
'Their reach should be extended to provide regular scrutiny of
regulators, executive agencies, quangos and the like.'

4. The chamber should remain central to accountability
'With space for more questions and short 'public interest' debate . . .
"in short, the chamber should be more responsive to issues of
public concern".'

5. Financial scrutiny should be central to accountability
'Financial scrutiny should be central to the work of the Commons
since it underpins all other forms of accountability.'

6. The House of Lords should complement the Commons
'The Lords has a significant role to play in the scrutiny of issues
which cross departmental boundaries.'

7. Parliament must communicate more effectively with the public
'Both Houses need to improve their communication with, and
responsiveness to, the public.'

(Hansard Society Commission 2001)

Agency governance

Under this proposal, the Secretary of State would appoint the chair
and other members of the NHS agency's board. All appointments would
be subject to the guidance and scrutiny of the Public Appointments
Commission. Board members would need experience and credibility
within the NHS. Crucially, the chair of the board would play a key role in

co-ordinating strategy and action between the agency and government. There are several different models for the boards of arm's-length bodies; in some, board members also serve a function in the strategic policy-making of the agency's host department. Such models would need to be reviewed in order to identify which is most appropriate for the NHS.

The board, with the approval of the Secretary of State, would appoint a chief executive, who would be able to speak independently of government on the role, management and performance of the NHS.

The agency would report at least annually to Parliament and be subject to regular review by parliamentary select committee. The chief executive would also have to provide an account of the agency's effectiveness to the Secretary of State, who has the power to dismiss any member of the board, including the chief executive. Its work would be brought under the jurisdiction of the parliamentary ombudsman.

The Secretary of State would be accountable for the effectiveness of the agency, for its targets and the framework within which it works, and for its funding. Guidance to non-departmental government public bodies is that 'the responsible Minister is accountable to Parliament for the degree of independence which an NDPB enjoys, for its usefulness as an instrument of government policy, and so ultimately for the overall effectiveness and efficiency with which it carries out its functions' (Cabinet Office 2000). The agency's chief executive would have ultimate accountability for delivery within the NHS, and Parliament could hold the chief executive directly to account for any issue relating to the performance of the service.

Domestic and international precedents

Across public services in the UK and abroad, organisations at arm's length from government play important roles. Some of them focus on regulation (such as the Commission for Health Improvement), some on allocating funds and assessing performance (such as the Higher Education Funding Council) and some on the management and delivery of services (such as HM Prison Service).

There are also organisations that undertake a mixture of governance, management, regulation and delivery. The Environment Agency, for example, manages the delivery of public services alongside providing a range of services directly to the public. The Housing Corporation funds housing associations, sets their performance targets and regulates them.

Examples from across the UK add to the body of evidence on how to take this proposal further. None provides an exact model for an agency that would meet the unique demands of the health care environment, but each merits closer examination to identify lessons that could apply to such an agency.

Internationally there is a similar mixture of different types of public bodies undertaking the funding, managing, regulating and delivery of public services. Many European governments define their role as setting national standards and frameworks for health care while devolving responsibility for management, regulation and delivery to others:

- In Finland, the centre focuses on steering the health care system by means of information, framework legislation and experimental projects. The Ministry of Social Affairs and Health issues framework legislation in health and social care policy and monitors implementation.
- In Sweden, the role of the minister is to ensure that the system runs efficiently and in accordance with fundamental objectives. The National Board of Health and Welfare acts as the government's central advisory and regulatory body.

- In Denmark, the central government plays a relatively limited role in health care, its main functions being to regulate, co-ordinate and advise.
- In Germany, decision-making is shared between the Länder and the federal government, and the powers governing statutory insurance schemes are delegated to non-governmental bodies.

Conclusion

Government and the NHS – Time for a New Relationship? has examined the case for an NHS agency. The idea is not new, but despite repeated expressions of interest, it has not been explored fully before. The analysis has shown what an agency could offer in the context of a health care system increasingly characterised by different forms of arm's length governance.

As we have seen, an NHS agency could allow greater parliamentary scrutiny, debate and accountability where government policy-making, the implementation of that policy and the performance of the health system are concerned. It could also help to increase NHS ownership of, and commitment to, delivering an agreed set of national standards and targets for long-term improvement.

However, this paper also acknowledges the conceptual and practical challenges posed by the agency model: specifically, the need to develop a new understanding of accountability that keeps national politicians at the heart of strategic decisions while allowing a non-elected agency chief executive to take responsibility for the implementation of policy and subsequent improvement of the health care system.

Some final comments on the analysis are offered under the following headings:
- the historical debate over an NHS agency
- the case for an NHS agency
- ways to test the relevance of the agency and take it forward.

The historical debate over an NHS agency

This paper has examined the debate about agency status since 1944, and has come to four conclusions.

■ First, the debate has followed a consistent pattern so far. Initial reactions to the proposal for an NHS agency have usually been positive, but stereotyped assumptions about accountability have soon led to its rejection. These include the following beliefs:
   – Public sector accountability runs in a direct and hierarchical fashion, without break points or thresholds, from individual health provider to Secretary of State.
   – The validity of any system of accountability should be judged by how far MPs (and by extension their constituents) are able to hold the Secretary of State responsible for any problem or grievance.
   – Parliament may only hold ministers and not civil servants (let alone the chief executives of arm's-length agencies) to account for their actions and achievements.

   Each of these assumptions has been challenged by the steady growth in arm's-length public bodies, together with the parallel evolution of parliamentary mechanisms for holding such bodies to account. This does not mean that the problem of accountability has become easier to address – rather that the traditional objections to the agency model are now less valid.

■ Second, each time during the history of the NHS that the idea of an agency has been considered, the motives for doing so have been different. Similarly, the successive rejections of the idea have been for different reasons. Each debate has considered different proposals in the context of a differently organised NHS, as a way of achieving different objectives.

The arguments for and against setting up a 'public corporation' to manage services across the country may not be relevant in the current environment where health care providers may apply for 'freedom' from central control. Instead, the present proposal goes with the flow of current thinking by aiming to reshape the national process for setting targets and implementing national policy in an increasingly diverse health care system, characterised by devolved governance and autonomy.

■ Third, the degree of political involvement in the NHS was acknowledged during the previous debates – and was considered an obstacle to harnessing the energies of local professionals and managers. Yet the way that politicians and the media are now constantly engaged in responding to an increased public appetite for news, opinion and response has made the inevitable involvement of national politicians in the fine details of health service delivery much more problematic. It has created a situation characterised by rapid policy development, leading to the threat of policy incoherence and to a perception among health professionals that the principles of subsidiarity and trust are being repeatedly breached.

■ Finally, one of the more influential arguments for rejecting an NHS agency now seems less valid than it was. Previously, the assertion that an arm's-length agency is inappropriate for 'politically sensitive' areas of service delivery had been widely accepted. However, this analysis considers the opposite notion that there are aspects of public services with high political risk that actually make agency status more appropriate. It certainly guarantees the high level of public, professional and parliamentary interest needed to ensure that national expectations are discussed more openly and that scrutiny and accountability over policy are improved.

The case for an NHS agency

The case for an NHS agency demonstrates the potential for enhancing the scrutiny as well as the implementation of policy, for developing parliamentary accountability for health care, and for increasing the ownership by NHS staff of national standards and targets, as well as their implementation. These benefits justify the effort involved in creating a new understanding of accountability, and new systems to make it work.

The continued building of Parliament's capacity to scrutinise both agency and government, and to hold them to account over health policy and its implementation is crucial. Parliament must be the basis of the new system of accountability that needs to be developed if a 'politically sensitive' agency at arm's length from government is to work.

The political environment that could accommodate an NHS agency is beginning to develop. Huge areas of public-sector activity are now being undertaken at arm's length from government, even in health. The commissioners, regulators and providers of health care are experiencing changes in status that seek to establish their freedom to act within certain national perimeters. The notion of separating the development of policy from its implementation is an application of the same logic: it is not as unthinkable as it once was.

The need to develop new structures of accountability is already being met by the greater willingness to place responsibilities for accountability on Parliament. This is reinforced by the greater willingness of Parliament to extend its remit to cover the non-department public bodies and executive agencies that are now at the heart of public service delivery. Although no existing arm's-length body offers an easily transferable model for an agency that would be dealing with the unique and complex undertakings of the NHS, the case for breaking new ground is strong and the environment highly conducive to success.

Ways forward

There should be wider debate about the agency model and its relevance to health care, particularly within Parliament and the political parties, and among health professionals.

Following this debate, a task force should be established to conduct a more formal review process of the criteria for agency status and its applicability to health care. This task force should be convened under the auspices of the Cabinet Office but include major stakeholders in health care, including representatives of government, the Department of Health, health care professions and the public.

Its terms of reference should include the following three specifics:
■ further review and analyse how such systems of devolved yet accountable governance are currently working
■ document those factors that seem to make existing arm's-length public bodies effective
■ fully explore the options for involving professionals and public in the work of an NHS agency.

The potential for an arm's-length NHS agency is one of a range of important, inter-linked issues shaping the future of our health service that need further research and analysis if decisions are to be based on sound evidence. The King's Fund will continue to contribute to wider debate, through research and publishing activities, and by hosting expert debates. Current activities includes research, publishing and events in the following related areas, as part of a wider programme of work, *Shaping the New NHS*:

- **The impacts of new forms of competition and choice** We are researching the impacts of the new fixed-price market in the NHS, looking at the implications and likely results of new financial flows, of allowing non-NHS providers to contract for NHS care, and of enhancing patient choice. In collaboration with a number of other organisations and academics, we are contributing to an evaluation of the London Patients' Choice Project.

- **The management of chronic care** We are researching how stronger market forces might best be applied to enhance the management of patients with multiple and chronic medical conditions, drawing on lessons learned from managed care organisations in the United States, with a major report to be published later in 2003.

- **The role of medical professionalism** We are researching how professionals might best be supported in order to respond to new challenges, such as stronger market incentives, with a discussion paper to be published in 2004.

- **Decentralisation and the 'new localism'** We are analysing whether attempts by government to decentralise power in the NHS, and to give the public more power in shaping health services locally, will improve provider responsiveness in ways that obviate the need for stronger market incentives.

See Linked publications (pp 54–6) for details of published and forthcoming *Shaping the New NHS* titles.

References

Appleby J, Coote A (2002). *Five-Year Health Check: A review of government health policy 1997–2002*. London: King's Fund.

Appleby J, Harrison A, Devlin N (2003b). *What is the Real Cost of More Patient Choice?* London: King's Fund.

Audit Commission (2003). *Health National Report: Achieving the NHS Plan*. Wetherby: Audit Commission Publications.

BBC website:
http://news.bbc.co.uk/hi/english/static/audio_video/programmes/breakfast_with_frost/transcripts/blair16.jan.txt

Cabinet Office (2003). *Public Bodies 2002*. Available at:
www.cabinet-office.gov.uk/agencies-publicbodies/publicbodies/index.shtm

Cabinet Office (2000). *Non-Departmental Public Bodies: A guide for departments*. London: Cabinet Office.

Commission for Health Improvement (2003). *Getting Better? A report on the NHS*. London: The Stationery Office.

Department of Health (2003). *Chief Executive's Report to the NHS 2002/03*. London: Department of Health.

Department of Health (1994). *Review of the Wider Department of Health*. London: Department of Health.

Department of Health (1993). *Managing the New NHS: A background document*. London: Department of Health.

Dixon J, Le Grand J, Smith P (2003a). *Can Market Forces be used for Good?* London: King's Fund.

Hansard Society Commission (2001). *The Challenge for Parliament: Making government accountable.* Report of the Hansard Society Commission on Parliamentary Scrutiny. London: Vacher Dod Publishing.

House of Commons Public Service Committee (1996). *Ministerial Accountability and Responsibility: Second report/public service committee.* London: HMSO.

King's Fund (2002). *The Future of the NHS: A framework for debate.* London: King's Fund.

Langlands A (2003). *Synchronising Higher Education and the NHS.* The Nuffield Trust. London: The Stationery Office.

Ministry of Health, Department of Health for Scotland (1944). *A National Health Service.* London: HM Stationery Office.

Ministry of Health, Secretary of State for Scotland (1957). *Report of the Committee of Enquiry into the Cost of the National Health Service.* London: HM Stationery Office.

National Audit Office (2000). *Good Practice in Performance Reporting in Executive Agencies and Non-Departmental Public Bodies.* London: The Stationery Office.

NHS Executive (1994). *Managing the New NHS: Functions and responsibilities.* London: Department of Health.

NHS Management Inquiry (1983). Leader of Inquiry: Roy Griffiths.

OECD (2002). *Distributed Public Governance: Agencies, authorities and other government bodies*. Paris: OECD.

The Office of Public Services Reform (2002). *Better Government Services: Executive agencies in the 21st century*. Available at: www.cabinet-office.gov.uk/agencies-publicbodies/ guiddepts/guidance3.shtm

Riddell P (2000). *Parliament under Blair*. Politico's Publishing.

Royal Commission on the National Health Service (1979). *Report*. London: HM Stationery Office.

Linked publications

We publish a wide range of resources on different aspects of the NHS.
See below for a selection. For the full range of our current titles, visit our
online bookshop at **www.kingsfund.org.uk/publications** or call Sales
and Information on **020 7307 2591**.

Shaping the New NHS: published titles

What is the Real Cost of More Patient Choice?
John Appleby, Anthony Harrison, Nancy Devlin

At first glance, more patient choice seems to be unequivocally 'a good
thing'. But what trade-offs are really involved – and what price are we
prepared to pay? How far can individual freedoms be extended while
still retaining the essential objectives of the NHS? This discussion paper
lays out the questions the Government must answer if it wants to place
patient choice at the heart of a taxpayer-funded health care system.
They include how extra costs will be met, whether patients are willing
and able to exercise choice in their own best interests, and what kinds
of limits to choice might be needed.

ISBN 185717 473 9 May 2003 52pp £6.50
Free download at www.kingsfund.org.uk/publications

Can Market Forces be Used for Good?
Jennifer Dixon, Julian Le Grand, Peter Smith

As the Government seeks to accelerate change in the NHS and make
services more responsive to public demands, the argument for market
disciplines versus planned provision is being hotly debated. This
discussion paper brings together the views of three seasoned
commentators. Julian Le Grand supports the introduction of stronger
market incentives to prompt improved performance among secondary

care providers, Peter Smith argues against even modest experimentation with stronger market incentives, and Jennifer Dixon asks whether it is possible to combine the best of market disciplines with planned provision.

ISBN 1 85717 477 1 March 2003 50pp £6.50
Free download at www.kingsfund.org.uk/publications

The Future of the NHS: A framework for debate

Should the Government be responsible for every 'dropped bedpan', or is it time for a decisive separation of political and managerial responsibilities? How can local responsiveness and innovation be supported alongside the drive for national standards? And can the extension of patient choice lever up quality? This paper, which brings together ideas from a group of commentators, academics and practitioners from health care and beyond, chaired by Lord Haskins, aims to stimulate the wider debate on which a reasoned, pragmatic consensus for the future depends.

January 2002 30pp Free
Free Download at www.kingsfund.org.uk/publications

Shaping the New NHS: forthcoming titles

How will Growing Pressures on Chronic Care be Managed?
Jennifer Dixon (ed)

How will the future NHS provide an effective response to growing demands for chronic care? Sharper market incentives – such as allowing funding to follow patient choice of provider, and encouraging more competition among providers, including those from the private sector – are being introduced. But these kinds of incentive seem more suitable for patients who are willing and able to travel to alternative providers for elective care, rather than patients who are old, frail and have complex chronic conditions. In the USA, managed care organisations offer excellent care for patients with chronic diseases in a competitive market. This paper asks what lessons the NHS can learn from their experience.

ISBN 1 85717 476 3 December 2003

What Future for Medical Professionalism?
Steve Dewar and Rebecca Rosen

Recent debates such as the proposed changes to GPs' and consultants' contracts have raised important questions about the rights and obligations of doctors. Are we witnessing a sea change in the old professional values on which the NHS was built, and will medical staff of the future work to a very different 'psychological contract'? This paper opens up the debate, and argues that greater clarity about the role of professionals will be crucial to a constructive discussion about the direction of health care reform and improving patient experience.

ISBN 1 85717 475 5 Spring 2004 £6.50
Free download at www.kingsfund.org.uk/publications

Other titles on the NHS

Claiming the Health Dividend: Unlocking the benefits of NHS spending
Anna Coote (ed)

The NHS is more than a provider of health services – it is the largest single organisation in the UK. How it recruits staff, procures food or constructs buildings affects the wider social, economic and environmental fabric of which it is part – which in turn affects people's health. This major report opens up an important debate about how the NHS might put its corporate muscle and spending power to work for health improvement and sustainable development – and how, in doing so, it can ensure it promotes health, as well as offering health care.

ISBN 1 85717 464 X May 2002 150pp £10.00
Download summary at www.kingsfund.org.uk/summaries

Five-year Health Check: A review of Government health policy 1997–2002
Anna Coote and John Appleby (eds)

When the Labour Government came to power in May 1997, it promised to 'save the NHS' by cutting waiting lists, improving service quality, raising spending, and reducing health inequalities. Five years on, this comprehensive report scrutinises progress against pledges made by the Government during its first term of office in areas such as funding, staffing, and quality of care. It argues that money alone – while crucial – will not build a new NHS, and that professional, motivated staff and a focus on wider health issues also have a key role to play.

ISBN 185717 463 1 April 2002 138pp £7.99

Hidden Assets: Values and decision-making in the NHS
Bill New and Julia Neuberger

What do values really mean for a modern, publicly owned health service? On what basis can staff and policy-makers resolve the inherent tensions between equally valid – but competing – priorities, such as equity of access and increased patient choice, or efficiency and effectiveness? Based on a series of King's Fund seminars with distinguished thinkers and practitioners from UK health circles and beyond, this publication combines analysis and case studies to show how values can successfully translate into health care provision, and argues that for values to 'live' as an organisational reality, trade-offs must be visible, managed and explicit.

ISBN 1 85717 458 5 2002 230pp £17.00

Making the Right Connections – The design and management of health care delivery
Anthony Harrison

In all areas of health care, there is a growing emphasis on ensuring that NHS services are designed and delivered with the needs of patients in mind. This publication argues that, while the development of more patient-centred services is clearly a good thing, it is important to understand how this will affect professional roles and ways of working in the NHS. It delves into the reasons behind today's problems in health care, analyses recent NHS reforms, and provides suggestions for improvement on the current situation.

ISBN 1 85717 440 2 2001 205pp £17.99

The NHS – Facing the future
Anthony Harrison and Jennifer Dixon

The NHS is under more pressure than ever before – from the public, the politicians and the media alike. This publication offers a wide-ranging examination of the modern health service, and some of the challenges it faces – such as new technology, an ageing population and rising consumer expectations. The authors argue that if the NHS is to survive in this new, more demanding environment, standing still is not an option, and suggests how the health service can equip itself for the future.

ISBN 185717 219 1 2000 342pp £17.99

What's Gone Wrong with Health Care? Challenges for the new millennium
Alison Hill (ed)

Demographic changes are placing huge new demands on the NHS. Today's health service needs to make a radical shift from working as a service designed primarily to treat acute and infectious diseases to one able to deal with complex, long-term diseases associated with an ageing population, such as diabetes and heart conditions. This publication looks beyond the funding issues to suggest constructive new ways of ways of providing health care in the 21st century.

ISBN 1 85717 425 9 2000 134pp £14.99

From Cradle to Grave
Geoffrey Rivett

Published to mark the 50th anniversary of the NHS, this publication
tells the extraordinary story of the health service. Based on discussions
with people who played a key role in shaping the NHS, it offers a
comprehensive overview of all the main landmarks – including
achievements and breakthroughs in medicine, nursing, hospital
development and primary health care – in a way that combines
both clinical and health management perspectives.

ISBN 185717 148 9 1998 528pp £12.50

King's Fund Information and Library Service
Call our specialist health and social care library on **020 7307 2568/9** for
free searches of its database and a range of literature about NHS issues,
as well as other topics.